First published in 2016 by Barrallier Books Pty Ltd,
trading as Echo Books

Registered Office: 35-37 Gordon Avenue, West Geelong, Victoria 3220, Australia.

www.echobooks.com.au

Copyright ©Bambi Staveley

National Library of Australia Cataloguing-in-Publication entry.

Creator: Staveley, Bambi, author.

Title: How to make thin hair fat : causes and solutions for unexpected thinning hair in women / Bambi Staveley.

ISBN: 9780994577801 (paperback)

Subjects: Hair--Care and hygiene. Women--Health and hygiene. Baldness--Treatment. Baldness--Prevention.

Dewey Number: 616.546

Book design by Peter Gamble, Graphic Design, Canberra.
Set in Garamond Premier Pro Light Display, 13/17 and Minerva Small Caps.

All rights reserved. No part of this book may be reproduced or transmitted in any form or by any means, electronic or mechanical, including photocopying, recording or by any information storage retrieval system, without the prior permission in writing from the author. The moral rights of the author have been asserted. The opinions of the author are her personal views only.

The ideas, suggestions and advice contained in this book may not work for everyone and do not constitute a replacement for medical advice. The reader must conduct their own due diligence and research.

www.echobooks.com.au

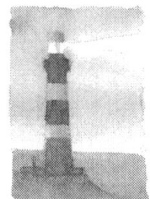

How to Make THIN HAIR FAT

Causes and solutions for unexpected thinning hair in women.

BAMBI STAVELEY

Contents

Introduction	ix
You are not alone	ix
Understanding Hair	1
Hair Growth Cycles	2
Normal vs Abnormal Hair Loss	5
Normal Hair Loss	5
Abnormal Hair Loss	7
Types of Hair Loss	9
Alopecia	9
Alopecia Areata	9
Female Androgenic Alopecia	11
Other Hair Loss Causes	11
Vitamins, Minerals and Hair Loss	15
Iron	16
Vitamin D	16
Zinc	16
B-complex Vitamins	17

Spotlight on Iron	19
How Will I Know if Low Iron is my Problem?	21
What Can I Do About Low Iron?	22
Will It Grow Back?	22
Dandruff, Dry Scalp and Hair Loss	23
The Follicles	23
The Scalp	24
Ageing Skin	26
Scalp Problems	27
Dandruff	28
Smoking	30
Stress and Hair Loss	33
Trichotillomania	37
Hair Dye and Hair Loss	39
Non-Physiological Causes of Hair Loss	43
Hair Washing	43
Heated Styling Products	44
Perming and Straightening	44
Hairsprays/Mousses/Gels	45
Biotin	47
What is Biotin?	47
How Much Biotin Do I Need?	48
Is There Such a Thing as Too Much Biotin?	49
Interesting Facts About Biotin	49
Can Diet Help?	51
Protein	51
Iron	52
Snacks	53
Natural vs Organic Haircare Products	55
Natural and Organic Shampoos and Conditioners	56

Chemical Shampoos and Conditioners	57
Think Twice About Keratin	**59**
Hairstyles for Thinning Hair	**63**
Going Platinum	63
Avoid a Straight Part	64
Shorter Hair Looks Thicker	64
The Blunt Cut	65
Avoid Back Combing	65
Use Hair Spray on your Roots	65
Tips for Summer	**67**
Sunscreen Cotton Bud	67
Rinse Hair in Fresh Water after Chlorine or Salt	68
Moisturise Hair – UV Protection Hair Care	68
Sun visor	68
Preventing Hair Loss	**69**
Is There a Cure?	**73**
Platelet Rich Plasma	73
Hair Plucking	77
Minoxidil	78
Propecia	79
The Trichologist	81
Hair Fibres a Cosmetic Solution	**83**
Conclusion	**89**
References	**93**

Introduction

You are not alone

You may have bought this book in a quest to find the answer to the sudden or gradual loss of your crowning glory. Or perhaps you have never had a thick head of hair and you are looking for ways to improve your hair health and thickness. Either way, you have come to the right place and I have much to share with you.

I suffered sudden, unexpected and visibly noticeable hair thinning in my forties as a result of a hormonal imbalance caused by surgery. This problem, perhaps seemingly small to some, changed my life in many subtle and some not-so subtle ways.

No doubt like you, I searched the Internet to answer my many questions.

Is this something that happens to other women? What has caused this? Is this permanent? Will it get worse? What can I do about it?

The answers were frustratingly lacking. Hair loss in men dominates the hair loss landscape; hair loss in women, although acknowledged, seems to have very little share of the online voice around the topic of hair loss.

During my many hours of online research into this phenomenon, I discovered that this problem for women, was on the rise. I learnt that women all over the world were suffering from thinning hair; yet I also discovered, to my horror, that most of the cosmetic solutions available were for men!

As a trained nurse with experience in mental health, I was acutely aware of the damage this kind of visible condition could do to a woman's self-esteem. Further, with many years in marketing and as an entrepreneur (an extremely rare combination of career choices and skills, I admit), not to mention my personal lived experience, I was fast realising my life was about to change.

The nurse in me knew I had to do something about this to help the millions of women I was now aware shared my plight; the entrepreneur in me saw an opportunity; and the marketing professional in me knew exactly what to do!

First and foremost, and like any nurse would do, I rolled up my sleeves and got to work to find a solution which could work for me and best of all, help others.

The fact that most of the cosmetic solutions available on the market had been developed for men was an interesting phenomenon. How often have we seen a cosmetic for men, let alone one where there wasn't really even a female equivalent?

Fast forward four years and my work has resulted in a women's hair loss blog, a range of cosmetic products designed specifically for women to provide instant relief to the problem, and now, this book.

Since setting up the Female Hair Loss Help blog and a business focused on products to help, I have fielded thousands of questions about hair loss from women of all ages and from all over the world. Sadly for many, their hair loss has been devastating and countless have given in to a life out of social circulation due to their acute embarrassment.

This book is about helping women with unexpected, sudden or gradual hair thinning and hair loss. In addition, for women suffering complete hair loss due to chemotherapy and the like, this book offers hope for thickening up regrowth when that time comes.

There is an enormous gap in the hair loss world (excuse the pun) of advice and products catering to women for whom hair thinning or hair loss is completely unexpected. So, as well as providing some suggested solutions, this book offers information for women who are trying to figure out what could be causing their hair to thin out, and provides some thoughts on what can be done about it.

It is no surprise that age plays a big part in the onset of thinning hair for many women, just as it does with men. However, my research uncovered a lot of other causes which, when combined with age and being female, can have a devastating effect on previously healthy hair.

All my research from the past few years has been compiled into this book to provide women with access to plenty of helpful information—all in one place.

There are so many possible causes for female hair loss, in fact the list is exhaustive. In this book I have covered the most common.

I hope that my research and suggestions will provide some relief for you and your hair loss problem and I really hope that you may soon be less stressed and less embarrassed.

I have personally thrived from the fabulous feedback from all the women who have tried my various solutions; the positive words of many get me through each busy day as my company and products are now helping women in more than twelve countries.

I wish you every happiness in your journey to healthier, thicker hair!

Bambi

Understanding Hair

The key to understanding why we might lose our hair is to understand how our hair functions in the first place. The human body grows three different types of hair: vellus hair, lanugo hair, and terminal or androgenic hair.

Vellus hair is the fine, downy hair (aka 'peach fuzz') that covers most of our body. Although it's usually almost invisible, it may be more visible on some people than on others, and may increase in visibility during puberty. It is 'designed' to help regulate our body temperature.

Lanugo hair is almost like a fine fur which covers babies in utero. Once a baby is born, lanugo hair becomes vellus hair. In some cases, lanugo hair may reappear later in life, for example, individuals with anorexia often grow lanugo hair.

Terminal or androgenic hair is the type of hair that you're probably most concerned about. Terminal hair is the hair on our heads, genitals and various other places on our bodies. This hair is usually visible, and unless mentioned otherwise, the type of hair we are focusing on in this book.

Terminal or androgenic hair grows in distinct cycles, and it is when these cycles are disrupted, affected or changed that we experience hair loss. The normal function of these cycles can be a result of many different variables, including genetics.

Hair Growth Cycles

Hair growth is cyclical, passing through three main phases: the growth phase (anagen), the rest phase (catagen), and finally, the shedding phase (telogen).

Anagen Phase

The anagen or 'growth' phase can last for two to six years depending on genetics. During this time, the cells in the root of each individual strand of hair are quickly dividing, and each hair will grow at the average rate of around 1 cm every 28 days. Interestingly, hair grows faster in summer than in winter!

Catagen Phase

The catagen, 'rest' or 'transitional' phase lasts for a few weeks after the anagen phase is finished. During this time, the hair follicle shrinks and cuts the hair off from its blood supply. The follicle pushes the disconnected hair closer to the surface of the skin as the follicle renews itself.

Telogen Phase

The telogen or 'shedding' phase can last anywhere from one to four months. During this time, some hair remains anchored to the follicle while not actually growing, yet others will fall out. At any one time, around 15% of your hair could be in the telogen phase. These are the hairs you see falling when you brush or wash your hair. Once a hair has been shed, the follicle will re-enter the anagen phase and re-commence the cycle.

Depending on the type of hair loss you have, this cycle is affected in some way either temporarily or permanently. For example, in hereditary hair loss, this cycle can become a lot quicker and it may take only months for a new hair to be shed—in some cases a new hair may not replace the recently shed hair at all.

Hair Growth Cycle

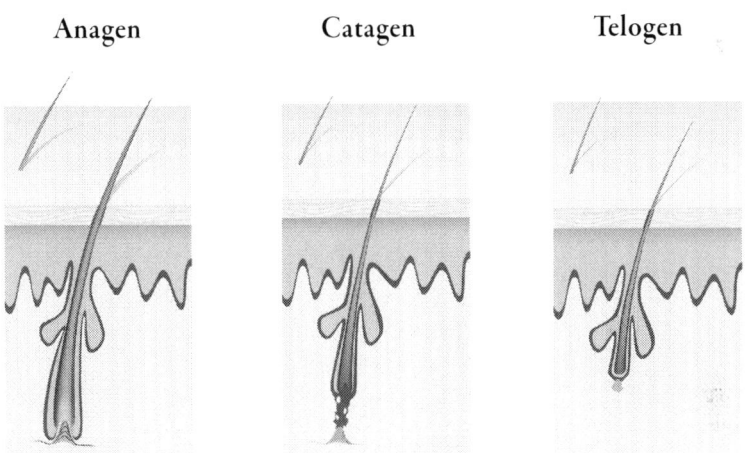

The three phases of the hair-growth cycle.

Normal vs Abnormal Hair Loss

Normal Hair Loss

It is normal to lose up to 100 hairs a day. In the previous chapter we discussed the normal cycle of hair growth and fall. Since all hair goes through this cycle of growth followed by a dormant stage followed by falling out, it makes sense that some hair will be falling out every day. So naturally we all notice some hair falling out every day or every other day, and it's perfectly normal for that to happen.

Seasonal Hair Loss

According to hair loss research in the United Kingdom, some women may also experience seasonal hair loss. That is, there is a time of year when more hair falls out than at other times of the year. You could be one of these people. I know I am.

It was when I was in my early forties that I first became aware of an unusual amount of hair fall. I decided to note it down in my diary as I had a suspicion that the same thing had happened once before and I wondered if it was a seasonal thing.

Sure enough, the same thing happened a year later. For me it was in autumn, or fall—aptly named for my circumstances!

Seasonal hair loss may be a sign of things to come, as it was in my case, or it can be nothing at all to be concerned about.

If you suspect that this could be you, write down the date when you first notice an increase in your hair falling out, then you may realise in a week or two you've forgotten about it, as I did for many years.

Then, if it happens again the following year, this will help you to isolate that you simply have a seasonal hair shed, which is likely to be perfectly normal for you.

Hair Washing and Brushing

When washing hair, it is normal to notice hair fall and this is when some people may become concerned. If you are someone who is trying to wash your hair less often to try to prevent it from falling out, then you may be continually frustrated that the hair fall is not reducing.

All day every day there are some strands of hair that have ceased to be attached, but they often don't appear or fall completely until you brush or wash your hair. The longer you leave it between washes the more hairs there will be in the fall stage, so there may appear to suddenly be more—when in fact, there isn't.

Over-washing, washing in hot water and washing using harsh chemicals can, however, cause your hair to dry out and break more easily. Make sure you're using good quality products, avoiding cheaper supermarket brands and conditioning adequately.

I have covered all these in later chapters.

Abnormal Hair Loss

Are you suddenly clogging the shower drain? If you suddenly notice an increase in the amount of hair loss in the shower, or in your brush, and none of the relatively 'normal' causes mentioned previously apply to you, then there are a few things you can do to determine if this is abnormal hair loss or just an unexplained deviation from normal.

Firstly, have a close look at the hair to determine if you can see the root of each individual strand of hair. The root looks like a tiny bulb wrapping around the end of the hair. Hair that has no root attached is likely to have broken off and although this is also a form of hair loss, breakage is a relatively simple problem to solve.

Note that hair loss due to chemotherapy and other potent drugs may result in hair fall that does not have the root attached.

If you do see roots in your fallen hair and you are sure that the amount of hair loss each day is consistently higher than normal, then it may be worth worth consulting a doctor to discuss some options. There are a number of blood tests that a doctor can order to test for common causes of hair loss in women and they may also refer you to a specialist.

Hair Loss in Patches

If you notice that your hair is thinning only in some areas and not in others, you may be experiencing the early stages of hair loss. If you're noticing circular patches of hair loss, you may have alopecia areata. If you see diffuse thinning (not localised) in the front of the head, the back of the head (or the crown) and the part line, you may have androgenic alopecia. Both of these are explained in full in the next chapter.

Scalp Discomfort

If you're losing more hair than usual and your hair loss is accompanied by a sore or itchy scalp, then you should seek medical advice as you may have a skin condition which is causing your hair to fall.

The good news about some scalp ailments that cause hair loss, is that when the scalp issue is resolved, hair usually grows back.

Hair Loss Accompanied by Other Symptoms

If you notice an increase in your hair loss and you also feel unwell or not your usual self in any way, there could be other issues worth checking with your healthcare professional. Common causes of hair loss include vitamin and mineral deficiencies that could leave you feeling run down and lethargic, so you may find that correcting these issues may not only stop your hair loss but make you feel a lot better in general.

Hair loss can also be a symptom of illness, especially auto-immune diseases, so the sooner you seek medical advice, the sooner you can address any health issues you may have, along with your hair loss.

Types of Hair Loss

Alopecia

Alopecia is the medical term for hair loss, so if you have some form of hair loss, whatever the cause, technically you have alopecia. Unlike the general perception of the term, however, this doesn't necessarily mean that you will end up completely bald. There are a few different forms of alopecia which vary depending on the type of hair loss and the cause

Alopecia Areata

Chances are that this is what's popping into your head when you think of the term alopecia. Alopecia areata is an autoimmune disease which can present in many forms.
- patchy hair loss all over the scalp (diffuse alopecia areata)
- complete baldness of the scalp (alopecia totalis)
- baldness in one area of the scalp (alopecia areata monolocularis)
- hair loss in multiple areas (alopecia areata multilocularis)
- total hair loss: head, face, body, pubic hair etc. (alopecia universalis)

Areas of hair loss in people with alopecia areata are usually well defined, rounded patches. Like most autoimmune diseases, it occurs due to the body's inability to differentiate between its own cells and foreign cells. This leads to the body attacking its own cells, in this case, the anagen hair follicles. Alopecia areata is quite rare (affecting 0.1 – 0.2% of people) so it's unlikely alopecia areata is the reason for your hair loss. However, you are more likely to have alopecia areata if you have other autoimmune diseases, or a family history of alopecia areata or other autoimmune diseases.

Thoroughly examine the pattern of your hair loss, and if you notice your hair loss is occurring in well defined, circular patches, you may, have alopecia areata. Get to your general practitioner (GP) for a professional opinion. Your GP may refer you to a specialist.

If it is determined that alopecia areata is the reason for your hair loss, don't fret! Often the condition will fix itself within a few months to a year. There are also medications (most commonly corticosteroids) that you can take to speed up the return of your hair. You may get flare ups from time to time, especially during periods of stress, so it's important to understand your hair loss causes and effects and manage these triggers as best as you can.

I can speak from personal experience here, as this happened to me some years before my diffuse hair loss. One day my hairdresser pointed out that there was a complete bald patch on the side of my head above my left ear. Interestingly, I didn't fret about it as it was hidden from view and to be honest, I completely forgot about it and it resolved itself within a few months.

However, as I mentioned earlier, this can, and in my case did, herald the possibility of future hair loss of a different kind, *androgenic alopecia*.

Female Androgenic Alopecia

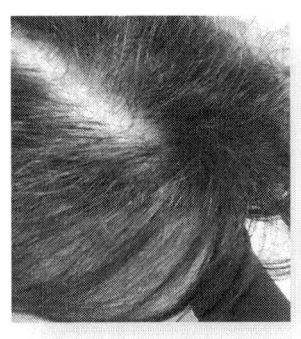

Androgenic alopecia is also known as female pattern baldness (yes, just like male pattern baldness, but don't worry, you're unlikely to experience as much hair loss as men do!). This actually *is* likely to be your problem and will affect more than 50% of women at some point in their life. If this is your problem, you will likely notice a widening part and/or thinning at the crown/back of your head.

A very common presentation is a widening part

A general health check may be a good idea at this point. There are some causes that can be determined by a blood test.

Other Hair Loss Causes

So, what if you don't have a form of alopecia? Why is your hair falling out? Well, there could be a number of reasons. The good news about the following is that they are usually temporary and reverse themselves in time.

Telogen Effluvium

Just like androgenic alopecia, *telogen effluvium* is really common. This occurs when your body has been through a period of stress. This could mean emotional stress like a divorce or losing your job, or it could mean physical stress like major surgery or dramatic weight loss or gain. Your hair is not a priority for your body, so as soon as you go through a stressful event and your body needs to be more strategic about assigning its resources, it soon ceases to consider growing hair as a necessity.

You may be thinking, 'well this isn't me, life's good at the moment". Well, as I explained earlier, your hair goes through various phases, so it may be weeks or even months until your hair reacts to your stress. The good news, if this is your problem, is that your body will likely regain its equilibrium on its own and your hair will return.

Post Pregnancy

Similar to telogen effluvium, this is all to do with those good old hair cycles! During pregnancy, higher levels of oestrogen prolong the hair's natural growth phase, which thereby prevents the hair's normal entry into the shedding phase. Many pregnant women comment on their luscious, thick hair when pregnant. However, after birth, these hormone levels fall, along with all that extra hair you were holding on to!

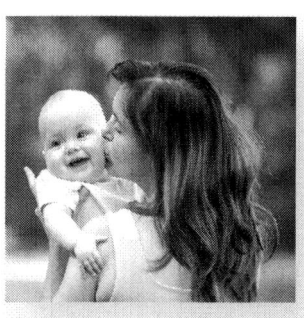

A widening part is usually the first sign that hair is thinning out post-pregnancy

For many women, especially those with naturally fine or thin hair, this post-pregnancy hair loss, can be quite distressing.

The good news is, that most women find that their hair returns to normal within a year. Some women find that they go through this experience with all of their pregnancies and some can be on their third or fourth pregnancy and experience it for the first time.

Menopause

Just like with pregnancy, menopausal hair loss is all about oestrogen levels. Ageing, which also brings about a drop in oestrogen, changes the density of our hair as well as the quality of our hair follicles. The bad news here is that, unlike post-pregnancy hair loss, postmenopausal hair is unlikely to return to its former glory.

But fear not; later in this book there are lots of ideas and solutions to help you deal with it. I've tried them all and, now that I have postmenopausal hair loss, I can honestly say that not a single soul can tell!

Even when I tell people what I do, they always say *'but you obviously don't have any hair loss, so how did you know this was a problem?'* Of course, I'm always thrilled when I hear that!

Polycystic Ovary Syndrome (PCOS)
(Also termed polycystic ovarian syndrome)

Although extra hair growth on the body is common in women with PCOS, in a cruel twist of fate, the hormonal imbalances associated with PCOS can also cause the hair on your scalp to thin. So, more hair where you don't want it and less hair where you do. Simply unfair!

Medication

Being prescribed a medication often indicates that a person is otherwise unwell, which in itself may be causing some hair loss. However, in some cases it could be the medication itself. It's important not to overlook any medications you may have been on long term, such as HRT or contraceptives, where you have altered your medication dosage or recently stopped taking them altogether.

Extreme Weight Changes

Restrictive diets of all shapes and sizes can result in a person missing out on various essential nutrients which, in turn, can cause hair fall. Likewise, gaining a significant amount of weight quickly can also put your body out of whack and under stress; this too, can cause hair to thin. So stay away from the fad diets if you don't want to lose more than just weight!

Illness

As I mentioned earlier, because hair is viewed by the body as non-essential, it is often the first thing the body stops assigning resources to, meaning it can begin to fall. Hair loss is a common symptom of a lot of illnesses e.g. autoimmune diseases, but what you may be surprised to learn is that even acute illnesses like gastroenteritis can put enough temporary stress on your body resulting in your hair beginning to fall out. The good news is that this type of hair loss will usually amend itself without intervention.

Vitamin and/or Mineral Deficiencies

This reason for hair loss is actually quite common in women. Like telogen effluvium, once deficiencies have been corrected, hair growth should return to normal on its own. I have outlined some of the most common vitamin and mineral deficiencies in the next few chapters.

Vitamins, Minerals and Hair Loss

You may have heard that taking certain vitamins can help slow or even stop hair loss. While this is true, it is unfortunately only true for some of us. If hair is falling due to a vitamin or mineral deficiency, then replacing the vitamin or mineral in our diet or through the use of supplements is likely to result in an improvement in hair quality and/or growth.

If, however, hair loss is not related to a deficiency, there is little proof that vitamin or mineral supplements will do anything to help. Despite this, some people without deficiencies swear by certain vitamins and minerals for hair loss.

Below is a quick rundown of the most common vitamins and minerals that *may* have an impact on hair loss. To determine whether any of these could be contributing to your problem, all you will need is a simple blood test.

But please take note, do not increase your intake of any vitamin or supplement without checking with your doctor first. While hair loss can be the result of a deficiency in some of these essential vitamins and minerals, there can be even greater adverse side effects from taking too many!

Iron

There has been a lot written about the connection between iron and hair loss so it's probably not a surprise to see it at the top of the list. Iron is an essential mineral for our bodies and is required for a number of different bodily functions, from immunity to the synthesis of DNA and the transmission of nerve signals. Iron is also a major component of haemoglobin, the red blood cells responsible for carrying oxygen in our blood. Iron is also an essential component of healthy hair.

If you suspect low iron might be contributing to your hair loss, you can read in greater detail the connection between low iron and hair loss in the following chapter 'Spotlight on Iron'.

Vitamin D

Low vitamin D is extremely common, especially if you're someone who doesn't spend much time in the sun. Vitamin D is important for the hair cycle, so it is possible that correcting low vitamin D could improve hair loss symptoms. Interestingly, having low vitamin D can also affect our ability to store iron, thus an extra reason for low vitamin D contributing to hair loss.

Zinc

It's quite easy to be low on zinc, especially if you sweat a lot. Zinc is required for a lot of essential bodily functions including cell reproduction and maintenance of hormone levels which can affect hair loss. Importantly, a zinc deficiency can also mean that you are not adequately absorbing other vitamins and minerals which in turn, may also cause hair loss! A zinc deficiency is also easy to spot through a blood test and easy to fix with supplements and/or diet changes. Bonus hint: chocolate is a good source of zinc, the darker the better—now you have an excuse!

B-COMPLEX VITAMINS

There is often a lot of talk about B vitamins and hair (especially biotin, which we will get to later), and it seems to crop up as the topic de jour for hair loss bloggers from time to time. B vitamins play an important role in the nervous system, in hormone regulation and in the immune system.

Many hair loss sufferers swear by B vitamins and believe that they have not only grown more hair, but that their hair is thicker and stronger.

Spotlight on Iron

As stated earlier, iron is an essential mineral for the body and is required for numerous bodily functions, such as immunity, synthesis of DNA, and the transmission of nerve signals. Iron is required for the creation of red blood cells and is also a major component of haemoglobin, the protein in the red blood cells that is responsible for carrying oxygen around in our blood. Iron is also an essential component of healthy hair.

You are possibly familiar with fatigue as a symptom of low iron. The reason for this is that serum ferritin (iron in your blood stream) carries oxygen around your body. Our cells need oxygen to function and with reduced ferritin comes reduced oxygen, and with reduced oxygen comes reduced function and exhaustion.

Iron is also an essential component of healthy hair as ferritin is needed in abundance by our hair follicles.

If low iron is your issue you will probably notice a telogen effluvium or diffuse type of hair loss, as discussed earlier. This is a condition where more than normal amounts of hair fall out, or shed. The overall appearance is of thin hair and often the first thing a woman notices with this type of hair loss is the sudden increased appearance of the scalp through the hair, or a much thinner ponytail.

This type of hair thinning can happen relatively quickly, but for some it can also happen very slowly over a period of years. Although this is observed in all age groups, it is the most common cause of hair loss in pre- and post-menopausal women.

To find out if your iron levels are low you will need to visit your general practitioner (GP) for a blood test. To test for low iron, your GP will likely order a couple of different tests: serum iron to see just how much iron is circulating around your blood stream; your ferritin levels to gauge the amount of iron stores you have; and other tests including red cell count and haemoglobin levels. These will provide an overall picture of your iron levels as a good starting point.

The reason low iron results in hair loss is because when the body is low in iron it uses less of its stores on non-essential processes such as maintaining and growing hair; rather concentrating its iron usage on life-sustaining essentials such as oxygen supply.

While low serum iron is certainly a factor in hair loss, once iron stores are depleted, the resultant hair loss can be even more devastating. A protein called ferritin stores iron for later use by the body. When ferritin stores in the hair follicles decline, the hair that is produced will often be dry, brittle, non-pigmented and fine. Because low iron stores deplete both the number of hairs on your head as well as their volume, it takes much longer for the body to recover. So if you suspect your iron levels are low, then get to your GP for some tests before your iron stores become affected too.

Iron is also important for the regular functioning of the immune system. Therefore, low iron can also lead to hair loss conditions like alopecia areata.

However, as I mentioned earlier, do not start to take an iron supplement based on your reading here or anywhere else. Too much iron can be dangerous and you should only take an iron supplement on the advice of your doctor.

How Will I Know if Low Iron is my Problem?

To be sure that you have low iron levels, you will need to visit your GP who will refer you for a blood test. However, here are some common symptoms of low iron levels which you may recognise.

- general fatigue
- weakness
- pale skin
- shortness of breath
- dizziness
- brittle nails
- tingling or a crawling feeling in the legs
- swelling or soreness in the tongue
- strange cravings for non-food items, such as dirt, ice and clay
- cold hands and feet
- fast or irregular heartbeat
- headaches

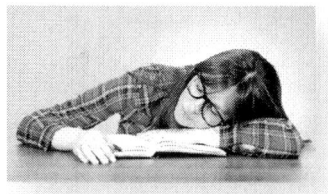

Low iron can result in general fatigue along with a hair-loss gap as seen here on the top of the head, around the part.

This is not an exhaustive list, and many of the symptoms listed can be attributed to other things, so see your GP to confirm that you have low iron before taking any supplements. As mentioned earlier, taking iron supplements when they are not needed can be very dangerous.

What Can I Do About Low Iron?

Your GP will give you some recommendations which may include iron supplements and diet changes. The good news is that where hair loss is the result of low iron levels, restoring iron levels will usually, noticeably improve hair health.

Will It Grow Back?

Yes, it definitely can! I am living proof. Be patient though, as it can take up to eighteen months for hair to regrow because iron levels need to be restored first before the body can begin to re-establish its focus on growing healthy hair.

The third occasion I noticed my hair falling out was because my iron stores became dangerously low. [The first time was a brief spell of alopecia which I described earlier, the second time was due to a hormone imbalance.]

Immediately after my GP had confirmed that my iron levels were dangerously low, I began taking supplements. It was a good eighteen months before I really saw thicker hair.

And five years later, I still take iron supplements, while having regular checks to ensure my iron levels are at a safe level.

So if this is your problem, there is hope!

But again I stress, do not take iron supplements without the advice of your doctor. Too much iron can be dangerous.

Dandruff, Dry Scalp and Hair Loss

To grow healthy hair, we need a healthy scalp. Much like our garden needs great soil to grow healthy plants, so too our hair needs a well moisturised and healthy scalp to maintain healthy hair follicles.

The Follicles

By now you know that our hair originates from the follicle which is found just under the skin surface all over the body (with the exception of the palms and soles of the feet). Hair follicles are made up of three essential structures: the dermal papilla, the hair 'matrix' and the hair shaft.

The matrix surrounds the papilla and is responsible for producing the keratin protein that makes up the bulk of the hair fibre. The matrix is also responsible for providing the melanin to give the hair, which would otherwise be transparent, its colour.

The papilla is found right at the base of the hair follicle and it plays the most important role in gathering the nutrients from the blood vessels and feeding the follicle. When there are not enough nutrients in the circulating blood for the papilla to extract, the process breaks down.

Nutritionists will often report corresponding poor hair health in individuals with deficiencies in certain vitamins and minerals, in particular, iron and the B group vitamins; biotin being the most written about of the B group when it comes to hair loss.

While we know that the speed and pattern of hair growth is generally dependent on genetics, age, gender and hormones, nutritional deficiencies and hormone fluctuations can have a negative effect on healthy hair. It's not surprising then, that a diet high in fast foods and lacking good balance will have a negative effect on our hair.

The Scalp

Just like the need for healthy follicles to produce healthy hair, we also rely on a healthy scalp to maintain healthy follicles.

Once again, good nutrition plays a major part in maintaining a healthy scalp. But significantly, quality hair care products are also important.

The scalp and all the skin on the body is made up of the dermis, the epidermis and subcutaneous tissue. And while much has been written about the hair follicle and its important role in healthy hair, to maintain healthy hair growth and the all-important, hair shaft thickness, the skin which houses the follicle must not be neglected.

Many studies have been carried out on hair transplants and there is a plethora of papers and research on the subject. One important factor in a successful hair transplant is the quality of the scalp tissue into which it is transplanted. Clearly a healthy intact hair follicle is also needed for the survival of the hair transplant, but studies have shown that even with a healthy follicle, if the scalp skin is not healthy or is damaged in some way, the follicle will struggle to grow. This can result in the growth of a thin and very fine hair shaft. Therefore it is both the skin and the follicle that play a crucial role in healthy hair growth.

There are many types of scalp health issues, some you can manage yourself, while others should be reviewed and managed in conjunction with a dermatologist. One utterly preventable scalp problem is caused by excessive sun exposure. As for all other skin on our body, the scalp can become sun burnt very quickly, and if you have thinning hair in particular, your scalp will have additional exposure. It is not easy to put sun-screen on our head, mixed in with hair, so we tend not to think of it.

Using a cotton bud to apply sun screen to thin areas or the part line is a good way to ensure you are not exacerbating a widening part by causing damage to that part of the scalp skin. But wearing a hat is obviously the most efficient sun protection there is! Some people believe that wearing a hat somehow causes rubbing or friction that in some way increases the amount of hair to fall out. Well, that is a complete myth! In fact, wearing a hat has the completely opposite effect.

Another option for women with longer hair is to wear your hair in a bun or ponytail when in the sun as this too will provide some protection for your scalp.

Protecting your scalp from the damaging UV rays of the sun is an absolute must if you want to maintain a healthy scalp for optimal hair growth.

Ageing Skin

As is unfortunately evident on the face, skin loses its elasticity with age. Skin also loses its density and becomes much thinner as we get older. This is also true of the skin on our scalp. So while our follicles reduce in size with age, thus producing a thinner hair shaft, and our scalp skin ages along with it, it would seem unlikely that our hair wouldn't also show signs of aging.

Sometimes it is a reduction in hair shaft thickness that is the first noticeable symptom of aging hair in a woman. For women with thick, dark-coloured hair in particular, where the hair shaft itself has been extremely thick and coarse, a thinner hair shaft may give the overall appearance of hair loss, when in fact it may not be so. It is simply that age has resulted in a thinner hair shaft, giving the overall appearance of less hair.

While there are some signs of age-related hair loss we cannot do anything about, we can at least do everything we can to look after the skin on our scalp.

It makes perfect sense that since it is generally accepted that good quality facial cream preserves the skin on the face for as long as possible, we also think about the skin on our scalp.

As a teenager I was taught to never put conditioner on the roots of my hair. I was taught to only apply conditioner to the ends of the hair and in fact, I read recently that conditioner should only be applied from the ears down – all very well, if your hair goes that far!

As we age, that old advice is no longer relevant unless you are someone with very oily hair and skin.

For the rest of us whose skin and hair has always been dry or is getting drier with age, we need to change the way we treat our scalp and hair in order to preserve its quality and hopefully its density for as long as possible.

Firstly, and most obviously, apply conditioner into all parts of your hair—not just the ends. And secondly, and possibly controversially for some women, apply a good quality oil to your scalp on a regular basis.

About once a month, I like to massage an oil through my hair on the night before I plan to wash it. Not so much oil that it seeps out all over the pillow, but just enough to moisturise the scalp and follicles. I know some women put a treatment in their hair overnight and sleep with their hair wrapped in a hair towel turban wrap. This is perhaps worth a try if your hair is very dry and frizzy.

If you are prepared to give an oil a go, there are a number of good quality oils on the market these days. Try an argan oil specifically formulated for hair, or a chemical free hair 'recovery oil'.

The good news about increasing the moisture on your scalp and therefore on your hair, is that if your hair loss is exacerbated by poor quality hair strands, then this oil treatment has the bonus effect of improving the quality of your hair.

I have very dry hair and skin so I also add a squirt of oil into my conditioner every third or fourth time I wash my hair.

Scalp Problems

There are literally dozens of skin diseases that can affect the scalp, from acne to dandruff, and from psoriasis to impetigo, herpes and melanoma. Other conditions that can affect the scalp are cradle cap, lupus and ringworm.

I would strongly suggest you see your doctor for a referral to a dermatologist if you suspect you have any of these. I have seen women with what may appear to be very minor skin irritations of the scalp resulting in significant hair loss, only to see them a year later after treatment by a dermatologist and their hair growth has returned to normal. I can't stress enough that having the health of your scalp looked at is a great idea!

Dandruff

Did you know that those troublesome flakes you see in your hair and on your shoulders from time to time may not be dandruff? It's far more common and far more likely to be caused by a dry scalp. Did you also know that treating a dry scalp with anti-dandruff shampoos can make it worse?

What is Dandruff?

Contrary to popular belief, dandruff is not actually caused by the skin on your scalp becoming dry. Dandruff is actually caused by an excess of sebum which accumulates on the scalp and leads to an overgrowth of yeast and occasionally fungi. This causes skin cells to shed more frequently giving you that 'fresh from a snowstorm' look. Unlike dry scalp, dandruff has a yellowish tint and is greasy rather than dry and flaky.

Like many hair and skin issues, dandruff can be caused by a number of different things. There may be a physical cause such as poor nutrition (especially a diet too high in fat, sugar and/or starches), hormones, heredity and scalp sensitivity. Dandruff can also be a by-product of stress, being generally run down, infrequent hair washing and misuse or excessive use of styling products.

Treatment

You would be familiar with the plethora of dandruff shampoos on the market. Well, these anti-dandruff shampoos have some fairly strong medicated ingredients in them designed to sweep all the gunk from your scalp and inhibit the regrowth of any nasties. These same ingredients will worsen a dry scalp so it's always best to know what the cause of your shoulder snowstorm is before picking a treatment option.

A lot of people mistakenly believe that it is best to avoid shampooing often when dandruff is present; however, it's actually the opposite! You need to keep the excess oil at bay so that yeast and fungi cannot proliferate. Washing every second day should be sufficient but if you're noticing that your scalp still seems oily, it's ok to wash every day with an anti-dandruff shampoo until the problem is back under control.

Dry Scalp

I referred to scalp health earlier, but here I am referring to the visible effects of a chronically dry scalp. As we know, dry skin can occur anywhere on the body, including the scalp. Chronic dry scalp is likely to be itchy and the flakes smaller, whiter and more brittle than dandruff flakes. As mentioned earlier, the scalp is also easily over-looked when it comes to sun protection, which can lead to a peeling scalp—often mistaken and subsequently mistreated as dandruff.

Back to our garden analogy, I often think of a dry scalp much like the cracked dry and parched earth often seen during a drought. Of course, nothing can grow in earth like that. Similarly, a dry scalp, lacking in natural oils and moisture, will struggle to keep hair follicles healthy, as described earlier.

If your visible flakes are really the result of a dry scalp, then there's lots you can do. For all the reasons mentioned earlier, you would now be aware that a dry scalp can be a contributing factor to hair loss. So it pays dividends if you can get it under control.

Make a concerted effort to change your hair management regimen. Here's a summary of the tips mentioned earlier:

- Use conditioner from root to tip
- Massage an oil into your scalp as part of your regular conditioning treatment and occasionally over night
- Protect your scalp from the sun.
- Look after your scalp and you will have thicker, more manageable hair along with no more of that embarrassing snowstorm.

Smoking:

Some of you may be surprised to find smoking mentioned here. Did you know that smoking is bad for your hair, or more importantly, your hair follicles? By now you know what that means.

An observational study carried out in Switzerland in 2003 found that there was a significant relationship between tobacco smoking and baldness. The mechanism by which smoking causes hair loss is related to the effects of the smoke (and not the nicotine, tobacco or the other chemicals) on the small blood vessels of the dermal papilla of the follicle. According to the study, the genotoxicants in cigarette smoke cause damage to the DNA of the hair follicle, as well as an imbalance in the tissue remodelling that occurs during the hair growth cycle. Other inflammatory processes which lead to follicular inflammation and fibrosis were also evident.

None of this should be surprising since we are familiar with the damage smoking does to the skin, causing premature aging. It has also long been associated with the early greying of hair.

Stress and Hair Loss

Stress is another common and often overlooked cause of hair loss in women.

When you picture stress induced hair loss, you might be thinking of someone running around trying to get their life together whilst literally tearing their hair out. What you may not know is that stress can actually trigger hair loss on its own – no pulling needed. Here are some of the questions I get asked most frequently.

How Does Stress Cause Hair loss?

Understanding the hair growth cycle that I covered in Chapter 1 is the key to understanding why we might lose our hair due to stress. You will recall that hair growth is cyclical, passing through three main stages: the growth phase (anagen), the rest phase (catagen) and finally, the shedding phase (telogen).

Under normal circumstances, we have an average of 100,000 hairs on our head and as mentioned previously, on average we shed around 100 of these a day. When something disrupts these cycles, like stress, the cycle can speed up, which may result in more hairs in the shedding stage, or follicles may not grow a new hair once a hair is shed.

This occurs because growing hair isn't really a priority for your body—it's not keeping you alive. If you're stressed, your body focuses on just keeping you going and neglects unimportant tasks such as keeping your hair healthy and plentiful.

What Constitutes Stress?

Stress is a very broad term, especially when it comes to hair loss. When it comes to stress causing hair loss, we're not just talking about *emotional* stress. *Physical* stress, such as gaining or losing a significant amount of weight, going through surgery or coping with illness, is just as important.

Like with a lot of things, the severity of the physical stress required to trigger hair loss will vary from person to person. Some people may not experience hair loss even after experiencing life-threatening illness, whist some people will actually suffer hair loss after a bad bout of gastroenteritis.

Emotional stress is similar in that some people are not as susceptible to the physical side effects of stress as others. Unlike physical stress, it is unlikely that you will experience hair loss due to acute low levels of stress like being late for work (unless your hair loss is due to something like trichotillomania or you are particularly vulnerable to hair loss). Emotional stress is more likely to cause hair loss in situations such as the death of a loved one or a messy divorce; even moving house can be particularly unsettling. Still, everyday stress can have other negative health effects, so if you feel stressed often, it's a good idea to discuss this with your GP.

How Long Does Hair Take to Recover After Stress?

Due to the cyclical nature of hair growth, hair loss due to stress is unlikely to become evident until a few months after the onset of the stress. Likewise, it will take a few months for the hair cycle to re-stabilise after a period of intense stress. Once the hair cycle has normalised, it will take a further few months to regrow hair in any areas that have become sparse. So, the short answer is: at least six months after you stop stressing.

How Can I Prevent Losing Hair Due to Stress?

Besides the obvious (don't get stressed!) the best thing to do is visit your GP to talk through some options to help you identify stressors in your life so that you can learn ways to cope with or even minimise them. They can also order blood tests to ensure that there is no underlying medical condition that could be contributing to your hair loss and/or stress.

How Can I Help my Hair Grow Back After Stress?

There's no miracle aid, unfortunately. Just be patient and adopt some healthy hair habits. There are many helpful healthy hair tips included in later chapters.

The aim is to maximise strength and reduce breakage. It may also be beneficial to switch to organic hair care products and take better care of your scalp.

Trichotillomania

What is Trichotillomania?

Trichotillomania is an impulse control disorder where the sufferer has an overwhelming urge to pull their hair out. Sufferers may pull out head hair, eye brows, eyelashes, beard hair or any other hair covering their body until they are visibly balding.

What Causes it?

Doctors are not sure what causes trichotillomania. Some studies believe that it is a form of addiction, whilst others believe it is more closely related to mental health conditions such as anxiety and depression.

Can it be Cured?

Many sufferers have shown improvement through psychotherapy and hypnosis; however, there is no known guaranteed cure yet.

What Should I do if I Think I Have it?

As with most of the other hair loss causes mentioned in this book, it's a good idea to visit your doctor. You may be given a referral to a psychologist or somebody who can help you get to the bottom of *why* you are hair pulling. There are also some great organisations that provide support and advice to sufferers of trichotillomania, a quick search on the Internet should bring up an organisation close to you.

Hair Dye and Hair Loss

I get asked by lots of women whether hair dyes could be causing their hair loss. Unfortunately, like most hair loss related questions, there is no simple answer. The short answer is: no, probably not, but maybe.

When we dye our hair, we are essentially dying something that is dead. Once the hair has reached the skin's surface, it no longer contains any living cells. Hair grows from the follicle at the root and is fed via the bloodstream. It is for this reason that many people assume that hair dyes cannot possibly cause hair loss and for the most part, that is true. However, there are some instances where hair dye *may* be the cause of, or at least a contributing factor to, hair loss, even though these instances are rare.

In some people, some hair dyes can penetrate the hair follicle itself and cause the follicle to die or become inactive. It is not known why this can happen to some people and not others. Some experts speculate that it may be an allergy or reaction to certain chemicals; others think it may have more to do with individual hair, skin and follicle types. It is important to note, however, that dying hair is extremely unlikely to be the reason for your hair loss.

But there are a few other factors with regard to hair dying that are worth mentioning.

It is possible that your hair may *appear* thinner if you are colouring it. If you are lightening your hair you are stripping out some of the pigment and nutrient from the surface of the hair shaft, making it finer, drier and more brittle. Brittle and dry hair tends to be more fickle and breaks more easily; both of these attributes lead to the appearance of less hair. Keep in mind also that lighter hair tends to look less dense.

If you are darkening your hair, then you are adding pigment to a hair shaft that otherwise is lacking pigment. Therefore, darker hair tends to look denser and hence, thicker.

If you have decided to lighten your hair as you age, then you may be noticing visibly thinner hair, not necessarily caused by hair loss, but by the simple phenomenon that lighter hair actually looks thinner.

Bear in mind that while darker hair may look thicker, it is also more likely to make thinning hair more noticeable for an entirely different reason. Dark hair is such a vastly different colour to the scalp in fair-skinned individuals, that the contrast between the hair and the scalp is more noticeable.

The visibility of the scalp through the hair is the number one embarrassing element mentioned by women suffering hair loss. It is for this reason that cotton hair fibre concealers like BOOSTnBLEND for women have become so popular. Their primary purpose is to thicken each strand of hair to obscure the visibility of the scalp.

Synthetic hair fibres come in a variety of colours and work by simply shaking them onto dry hair to add extra volume at the roots. This extra volume at the roots eliminates the contrast between dark hair and light scalp so that visible hair loss completely vanishes.

Minimising Exposure to Hair Dye

If you have been tested for all the usual culprits and still have not found a reason for your hair loss, the only way to determine that your hair dye is the culprit is to stop dying it for at least a few months to see if your hair loss eases.

This may be out of the question for many of us, though, so here are some tips to minimise the risk.

- Find a salon that uses natural (or mostly natural) dyes. When hair dyes have been found to be the culprit for hair loss, it is usually a specific chemical or combination of chemicals used in the dye, rather than the act of dying itself. If you tend to be sensitive to chemicals or have sensitive skin, it's a good idea to stay away from chemical hair products too.

- Consider 'off-scalp' hair colouring. The use of foils is a good way to colour your hair without slathering the hair colour on your scalp. Foils and tips can give the overall appearance of a different colour without the need for hair dye to come in contact with your scalp. Try highlighting to lighten hair all over or lowlighting to darken hair.

- Use natural and/or organic hair products. Just like with hair dye, slathering your scalp with chemical laden shampoos, conditioners and styling products can not only be harmful but is completely unnecessary. There are plenty of organic hair care products on the market these days, and many women report that switching to these products has given them much stronger and healthier hair, which means less breakage. I have covered further information on the benefits of switching to organic hair products in a later chapter called 'Natural vs Organic Haircare Products'.

Non-Physiological Causes of Hair Loss

Hair loss isn't always caused by one of the physiological changes I've mentioned. Sometimes, you might just be mistreating your hair without even knowing it, leading to breakage and poor quality hair.

Hair Washing

Washing hair too frequently can lead to a reduction in the sebum necessary to keep hair healthy and hydrated. By constantly washing away this natural moisturiser, hair can easily become dry and brittle and may be susceptible to breaking more easily. If you suspect this is you, then try to cut down on washing your hair and make sure to use good quality shampoos and conditioners to nourish your hair.

It's also a good idea to wash your hair in cooler water as hot water can further damage your hair and scalp. If you are a woman who is concerned about the skin on your face becoming prematurely wrinkled, then you may have read that you should never wash your face in really hot water and particularly avoid running it under the hot water in the shower. Perhaps by now you are beginning to see that there is a connection between healthy hair and the condition of your scalp. So it stands to reason that keeping your scalp from the potential destruction caused by very hot water makes perfect sense!

Heated Styling Products

Hair dryers, hot rollers, curling wands and hair straighteners are notorious for causing hair breakage. The excessive heat used to change the shape of your hair also dries and fries it at the same time. If you must use heated styling products, load up on a good quality moisturising conditioner and use a leave-in moisturiser as well. Some companies also make heat protection sprays but the jury's still out on whether these sprays really do much to protect your hair from heat damage.

Perming and Straightening

Do you know every aspect of your hair dresser's life back to front? If so, you may be visiting too often! Most of us are aware that the chemical preparations used by hairdressers to alter the look of our hair are usually not good for the overall quality of our hair. Perming and straightening solutions have definitely improved over the years and don't 'cook' our hair like they did in the '80s; however, they do still dry hair and cause it to become more brittle, leading to hair loss.

If you really can't live with your hair as it is, consider spending the extra money and get an intensive hair treatment each time you go to the salon.

Hairsprays/Mousses/Gels

Loading up on styling products to get your look just right can be harmful to fine, weak hair. Whilst light use of your favourite product should be fine, going overboard can dehydrate and weaken hair. Stay away from really heavy gels that cause hair to become super sticky; instead, opt for lighter, moisturising hair sprays and mousses. Further, avoid brushing out styling products as you are likely to cause a lot of hair breakage that way. Instead, gently wash out your products in the shower and if you still have some tangles remaining, use a wide-toothed comb to apply conditioner throughout the hair. This will minimise the damage and breakage from trying to brush knots out of dry, brittle hair.

What Can I Do if My Hair is Dry and Breaking?

If all this talk of dry hair is sounding familiar, there are a few other things you can do in addition to those mentioned above:

1. Between your shampoo and conditioner, towel dry your hair. You would know that if you are trying to apply face cream to a wet face that it won't be well absorbed—the same applies for your hair.

2. Use the hair dryer to partially dry your hair before applying your styling products. For the same reason as tip #1.

3. Resist the temptation to rub your hair vigorously when towel drying. You can do a lot of damage to wet hair as it is more likely to stretch and break. Blot and dab! Try a specially designed microfibre hair towel wrap for women with thinning hair.

4. Never brush or use a fine-tooth comb on wet hair. Wet hair is slightly elastic and can break very easily. Always use a broad-tooth comb and be gentle with wet hair.

5. Never put your hair into a ponytail when it is wet, especially not a tight ponytail. For the same reason as tip #3 and tip #4, pulling it up tightly into a ponytail or into rollers or curlers when wet, can also cause the hair to break.

6. Avoid sleeping in rollers. As you can imagine, rollers or curlers put a huge amount of stress on the hair. I probably don't even need to mention now that doing so to wet hair in particular, is a definite no-no.

Biotin

If you've done a bit of Internet research about hair loss, you've probably heard about biotin, a so-called 'miracle' cure for hair loss, and you're probably wondering why it hasn't made an appearance in this book so far. Well read on and potentially save yourself a lot of wasted hope, money and some horrible side effects.

There are no scientific studies to suggest that someone with hair loss, not due to a biotin deficiency, will see any improvement in their condition by consuming biotin supplements. It's also worth remembering that you should NEVER start taking supplements on your own—see your GP first to be tested and advised on what you may be deficient in. After all, there's no point in taking something that you don't need!

What is Biotin?

Biotin is a B-complex vitamin; you may also have seen it referred to as Vitamin H. Like all B group vitamins, biotin is water soluble, so your body doesn't store it. This has led many to assume that we need to be constantly bombarding our bodies with biotin supplements, but this is simply not the case. Biotin can be made in the intestine and is also found in a huge variety of food, which is why biotin deficiencies are extremely rare.

Biotin is found in dairy products, egg yolks, oily fish (such as sardines, salmon and tuna), nuts (pecans, almonds, peanuts, walnuts), soybeans, legumes (beans, black-eyed peas), chicken and liver. It is also prevalent in fruit and vegetables including bananas, mushrooms and cauliflower as well as in whole grains and brewer's yeast.

So as you can see, anyone with a healthy diet is very likely to have sufficient biotin in their system.

How Much Biotin Do I Need?

While it is true that biotin plays an important role in the health of your hair, as we have just seen, most adults are likely to be getting enough biotin naturally and therefore would not benefit from taking a biotin supplement. In fact, many people have experienced some pretty nasty side effects due to the massive doses of biotin available on the market.

For example, a non-breastfeeding adult only requires 30 micrograms (mcg) daily (35 mcg for those breastfeeding) and the supplements found on the shelves range from 300 mcg to whopping 10,000 mcg, with the most common dose being 5,000 mcg! Furthermore, many of these companies suggest taking one tablet twice a day!

Many people don't believe there is anything wrong with taking a large amount of supplements, presumably because they are perceived as 'healthy'; however, you can cause yourself a lot of problems by taking supplements without the supervision of your doctor.

Is There Such a Thing as Too Much Biotin?

Biotin negatively interacts with the body's ability to absorb both zinc and vitamin B5 (aka pantothenic acid), which means that taking excessive amounts of Biotin can cause a deficiency in one or both of these elements. If you've been reading carefully, you might remember that a potential side effect of a zinc deficiency is hair loss! Guess what a potential side effect of a B5 deficiency is? Hair Loss! So you will actually risk worsening your hair loss by taking the massive amounts of biotin available on the market. Even if you are deficient in biotin, you don't need to be taking thousands of micrograms.

Another common side effect of taking biotin is acne which occurs due to the lowering of your B5 levels. Some bloggers (yes, bloggers, not doctors!) have suggested that taking B5 in conjunction with biotin alleviated their acne; however, many have wished they just never tried biotin in the first place.

In summary, the bad news about biotin is that it is probably not going to cure your hair loss and may actually make your hair loss worse and harm you in other ways. If you suspect that you may be deficient in biotin, see your doctor for a blood test. Your doctor will then be able to give you proper advice on the recommended dose for your needs.

Interesting Facts About Biotin

When biotin is taken at the same time as vitamin B5, there is some evidence to suggest that each diminishes the effectiveness of the other. The reason for this is that each of these inhibits the body's ability to absorb the other.

Raw egg whites bind with biotin in the small intestine and prevent it from being absorbed. Eating 2 or more raw egg whites a day over several months can lead to a biotin deficiency.

Alcohol is known to reduce the body's absorption of the B group vitamins.

Other symptoms of biotin deficiency include dry scaly skin, cracking in the corners of the mouth (called cheilitis), swollen and painful tongue, dry eyes, loss of appetite, fatigue, insomnia and depression.

Can Diet Help?

Diet is one of the first places you should look to improve your hair, skin and nails. You've heard the adage, 'You are what you eat'—but have you ever considered 'You are what you absorb'?

Many of us have digestive system and gut problems that can lead to the lack of absorption of vital nutrients. This was something that happened to me. A malabsorption issue was the cause of my dangerously low iron. If you think this could be you, then check in with your doctor.

A healthy gut as well as a healthy diet is important for healthy hair.

Protein

Do you get enough protein from your diet? Many women are not eating enough protein and since your body needs protein to make hair strong, you may find that adding a protein powder to your daily regimen or increasing your general protein intake may help keep your hair in healthier shape.

Summon up the usual suspects—meat, fish and eggs. If you are vegetarian, be sure to include at least the daily recommended amount of protein from other sources such as legumes and nuts.

Did you know that some of the most common dietary proteins also have other beneficial effects on our hair?

- **Milk** is not only a source of protein, but also a primary source of calcium which is needed for Vitamin D absorption. As mentioned earlier, recent studies have begun to uncover a link between low vitamin D and hair loss in women. Vitamin D has many other protective benefits too, so it may be worth having your levels checked if you think you could be lacking.
- **Eggs** are also a great source of protein and vitamin D, as well as B-complex vitamins believed to be involved in the development of keratin.
- **Salmon** is a source of protein and biotin, and has other important benefits as well. Oily fish such as salmon contain omega-3 fatty acids which we all know we need to include in a healthy diet, but did you know of its effect on your hair? Omega-3 fatty acids are vital for healthy, well moisturised skin and since our scalp is the skin that contains our hair follicles, it makes perfect sense that an unhealthy scalp will contribute to unhealthy hair.

Iron

As you've already read, iron is a fairly common cause of hair loss. Red meat is a good source of iron but if you're vegetarian or don't eat red meat, there are lots of other good sources of iron too. Vegetarians may need to keep a closer eye on their iron levels, however, as the type of iron found in plants is not as readily absorbed as the type of iron found in meat. Try to eat more green leafy vegetables, legumes (especially white beans and lentils) and quinoa, to name but a few sources. Vitamin C helps to absorb iron too, so eating foods rich in vitamin C with foods rich in iron is a great idea.

Snacks

Although many of us try to minimise our snacking, there are some good snacks from which we could really reap the benefits. Almonds are a great source of natural protein that can ease hunger at the same time. Since they contain magnesium there's an added benefit: magnesium is a great anti-stress mineral and for many of us, thinning hair is caused or exacerbated by stress.

While we are on the topic of stress, did you know that foods high in antioxidants also help to minimise the *effects* of stress. Try blueberries as a great source of antioxidants, as well as the daily recommended quantity of red wine (but remember, a high amount of red wine in our diets has the opposite effect!).

In addition to considering your diet choices, why not gear yourself up to also try some anti-stress mechanisms, such as yoga, going for a walk, stretching or hitting the gym?

Natural vs Organic Haircare Products

Could your shampoo be contributing to your hair loss?

It's no secret that being more active and closely scrutinising the chemical additives we put INTO our bodies is beneficial to our health; however, many of us are forgetting to pay attention to the chemicals we put ON our bodies.

A few years ago, mineral make up was all the rage for those looking for natural alternatives to the chemical gunk that we'd been slathering on our faces for decades. More recently, the health spotlight has been turned to the haircare market.

According to a recent survey of GPs, 64% said they had noticed an increase in female hair loss complaints in the last five years, which is likely to have contributed to this latest healthy haircare boom. But what are natural haircare products and are they worth the switch?

To quote one of the lovely ladies who wrote to me after trying an organic range:

> My hair has completely changed since I started using the [chemical free] shampoos and conditioners available from BoostnBlend. It's so much healthier, stronger and I notice a lot less hair fall in the shower when I wash it.

It actually has some shape now and I feel much less self-conscious about any visible scalp or my hair looking a bit dirty when it was freshly washed (anyone with flat, limp hair knows how that feels).

Yep. We sure do!

Natural and Organic Shampoos and Conditioners

Unlike most of the supermarket offerings, the newer, natural, organic shampoos and conditioners use essential oils along with plant and herb extracts to naturally cleanse and nourish hair without having to expose it to damaging chemicals.

Here I have listed some of the positive and the negative aspects of both chemical-free and chemical-laden shampoos and conditioners to help you make up your mind:

Positive:

- Safe for everyday and every other day use
- No harmful chemicals
- Won't strip the hair of natural oils
- Won't interact with or strip synthetic hair colours
- Won't dry hair out and make it brittle and susceptible to breakage
- Safe for use on all hair types
- Safe for use by the whole family, children and pregnant or breastfeeding mothers included
- Usually smell AMAZING!

Negative:

- Can be difficult to lather without the chemical sodium lauryl sulfate which is contained in most common shampoos
- Often more expensive.

Chemical Shampoos and Conditioners

Here I am referring to the supermarket and chemist brands. They use chemical cleaning agents to clean the hair, some of which can cause problems in susceptible people. They also contain a chemical called sodium lauryl sulfate which has been linked with a decline in the hair growth cycle.

Positive:

- Easy to lather
- Effective cleaning power
- Can be very cheap

Negative:

- Contain sodium lauryl sulfate
- Often harmful to hair with regular use
- Strips hair of natural moisture which can cause breakage, i.e. there is such a thing as 'too clean'!
- Chemicals can irritate the scalp contributing to or exacerbating issues like dermatitis, dandruff and dry scalp.

It is well worth your time to search for the organic products that are right for you. Read the ingredients lists, it will astound you!

Think Twice About Keratin

Is keratin good or bad for already thinning hair?

There has been a lot of buzz about keratin in the hair loss industry. It's been touted as a miracle product, able to smooth curls and frizz whilst adding body and shine. But is it really all it's cracked up to be?

The advertising and marketing of some hair products would have us believe that the keratin used in hair products like keratin hair fibres, keratin smoothing treatments and keratin shampoos/conditioners is the same 'keratin' that makes up our hair and nails.

Whilst this is almost true, and without getting too technical, keratin is actually a family of fibrous structural proteins, and humans have 54 functioning keratin genes. Only some of these keratin genes are found in human hair and they are not likely to be the same keratins found in hair products.

So where does this 'keratin' come from?

As well as being present in human hair, keratin is also found throughout the animal kingdom in wool, horns, feathers, claws and hooves. It is from these sources that most keratin hair product manufacturers synthesise their keratin. So whilst you may believe that you are buying something that closely resembles or imitates human hair, you are likely to be buying animal products.

If you are not a vegetarian does this really matter?

Well that depends. Synthesising keratin from animal parts makes keratin an 'animal protein' which means it naturally contains a large amount of bacteria. In order to turn the animal protein into a safe cosmetic product, significant amounts of bactericides and preservatives are required. Enter...more chemicals.

Are all keratin hair products made from animal protein?

No, not all of them, but most of them. Unfortunately, the products which are not made from animal protein aren't any healthier. The other way to 'make keratin' is to mix chemicals to imitate the structure of the forms of keratin found in human hair. These types of 'keratin' products are purely chemical concoctions rather than natural products.

But are keratin hair products really harmful?

No. Not in the main. However, if you notice any concerning changes in your health while using keratin hair products, it would be a good idea to mention it to your doctor. If you are someone who reads hair loss forums, you may have seen some people reporting side effects such as breathing difficulties and skin and eye irritations. These are extremely rare. The main chemicals to watch out for in keratin hair products are ammonium chloride and formaldehyde. Both are commonly used in keratin hair products and both are known to be harmful, even in small quantities, to some people.

Is there a way to boost natural keratin stores?

As keratin is a protein, you may find that increasing the protein in your diet may assist in preventing or slowing hair loss. As mentioned earlier, recent studies have suggested that women are not eating enough protein; since your body needs protein to make hair strong, a lack of it may be contributing to fine, thin or thinning hair. See the later chapter called, 'Can Diet Help?'

But what if you are using keratin hair fibres, are there any alternatives?

Sure! There are a few companies making hair fibres from cotton, rather than keratin. Since cotton fibres are plant based, rather than animal based, they don't require any chemicals so should be safe even for sensitive people. Most online reviews suggest that the cotton products have more positives than just the health and environmental benefits too, so you may find you prefer them anyway.

You will find hair fibres like BOOSTnBLEND for women are made from 100% natural cotton with not one keratin hair fibre in sight.

Hairstyles for Thinning Hair

Going Platinum

Platinum hair trends come and go, but it's not just for models or celebrities.

While many celebrities are embracing platinum just to stay on trend, there are some savvy women who have cottoned on to the advantages of platinum hair and they couldn't be happier.

Think about going platinum if you're going/are grey

It can be time consuming, expensive and just downright annoying to constantly dye away your grey roots, but if you have darker hair, they're simply too visible to ignore. It is well worth considering turning to the freedom of platinum coloured hair. Greys will blend seamlessly into this super on-trend hair colour and you can neglect the salon for long periods of time without looking like you're neglecting the salon. Pure genius!

Think about going platinum if your hair is thin/thinning

If you have light coloured skin and have thin or thinning hair, you would probably be aware that your scalp is often visible through your hair. You've probably used endless styling products and tried various hairstyles to hide that pink or lily white scalp skin. Here's where the skin hiding genius of platinum hair comes into play.

Platinum hair is much closer to your skin colour than, say, dark brown hair, so the lack of contrast between your scalp and platinum blonde hair will make your scalp much less obvious. Pair this with a platinum hair fibre concealer and you'll have thicker, on-trend hair with no visible scalp to worry about.

Avoid a Straight Part

So often we notice a woman with a thinning hair problem because she parts her hair in a straight line. The straight line makes the hair gap appear wider than it really is in women with thinning hair. It is likely you have seen the zigzag part used by many famous women in magazines on a regular basis. Well, zigzag parts are not just for the famous! You can easily do it yourself.

Play around with your part and work out what works best for you. If you are using hair fibres, apply a little on your usual part line. Then using a comb, make your zigzag before applying a bit more. Use your fingers to pat or fluff it in, and you're guaranteed to have much less scalp showing!

Shorter Hair Looks Thicker

From time to time women send me photos of their thinning hair and the first thing I often notice, it is just too long. We know and understand that if your hair is thinning, you want to give the impression of more hair. It might appear that longer hair gives the impression of thicker hair, but in fact, it is usually the opposite. When thinning hair is long, it tends to do two things to make the problem appear worse. First, because of the extra weight, it drags hair downwards so it tends to sit closer to the top of the head, exposing the scalp. Second, if hair is thin throughout, then the visual effect of long, thin hair gives a more obvious, overall impression of thin hair.

Try going for a shorter style and once your hair is lighter it will make it easier to lift your hair away from your scalp. Then apply a hair fibre concealer to your hair near your scalp and with less weight and less of the drag effect, your hair will appear thicker.

The Blunt Cut

It should come as no surprise to hear that a blunt hair cut gives the impression of thicker hair. The reason for this is that all your hair is ended sharply in one straight line. When thin hair is layered, it can make it look thinner at the ends. Give a blunt cut a try the next time you feel like a change.

Avoid Back Combing

Back combing or teasing your hair at the roots does have the effect of lifting your hair and with some hair fibre concealer it will appear thicker. But just be careful with back combing because if your hair tends to fall out, heavy back combing over a long period of time can make the problem worse.

Use Hair Spray on your Roots

After applying your hair fibre concealer, using one hand, lift your hair at the roots and spray under the hair with a firm hold hairspray. This slight lift can help to keep your hair looking bouncy and will also assist to keep your style camera-ready all day long.

Take note of later comments on the over-use of hair styling products and aim for a balance.

Tips For Summer

During summer our hair can take quite a beating! Here are some quick tips to help you survive summer with thin or thinning hair.

Sunscreen Cotton Bud

Many of us have a widening part or visible scalp and whilst we may be aware of the aesthetic drawbacks of this, we may not have thought about the potential health consequences. One of the key roles our hair plays is protecting our skin from the sun, so any areas not fully covered by hair are at risk of sun damage. It's a good idea to wear a hat whenever possible or tie your hair up to cover the gaps; however, these two looks may not be what we had in mind for that summer BBQ! So, a quick tip: apply sunscreen to a cotton bud and carefully apply sunscreen to areas of visible scalp. This will protect you against harsh UV rays without making your hair greasy. Of course, making sure you have a good coverage of a hair fibre concealer, along with a zigzag part line will also provide some protection!

Rinse Hair in Fresh Water after Chlorine or Salt

Spending time cooling off in the pool or at the beach is one of the best things about summer; however, our hair may not agree. Both salt water and chlorinated water can dry hair out and lead to breakage. An easy way to avoid this is, of course, to swim without getting your hair wet, but that's not always possible or preferable. If you get your hair wet, just rinse with fresh water to get rid of that drying pool or ocean water.

Moisturise Hair – UV Protection Hair Care

Between the extra sun exposure, the pool and the surf, our hair has the potential to get quite dry during summer. To protect against unnecessary breakage caused by dry and brittle hair, stock up on good quality treatments and leave-in conditioners to minimise breakage. Some hair care companies also make UV protection sprays that may help too.

Sun Visor

If you want to wear a hat to protect your face, but want to avoid hat hair, a sun visor is an excellent option! It also has the added bonus of covering any thinning areas toward the front of your head. Just remember to use the cotton bud idea from tip 1 if you go with the visor look!

Preventing Hair Loss

While it may sound unbelievable and too good to be true, if you are a woman who is aware of the predisposition for female hair loss in your family, then there may be a few things you can do to minimise the likelihood of the problem coming your way. Likewise, if you are suffering from hair loss and you have daughters, then this is great advice you can pass on to them.

Vitamins and Diet

You know that saying, 'You only get out what you put in"? Well as you have already read here, it applies to the health of your hair just as much as working hard in your career or when hitting the gym.

In order to have healthy hair, it's important to have a healthy body. There are countless vitamins and minerals that are essential for healthy hair—a deficiency in any one of them can cause hair fall. I have covered these in earlier chapters. However, it's important never to guess what you may be deficient in, as taking anything you don't need can be harmful. Visit your GP for advice.

As well as ensuring that you are getting enough vitamins and minerals, there are a few foods covered in the chapter called 'Can Diet Help' that you should make sure to include in your regular diet to help stop the onset of preventable hair loss.

Get Regular Blood Tests and General Checkups

It's pretty hard to know if you're deficient in anything if you don't get a blood test! Healthy individuals under 35 should get a blood test every 2-3 years, whilst those over 35 or with any known illnesses or deficiencies should get a blood test annually.

If you are worried about hair loss, mention this to your GP as this will ensure the correct tests are ordered.

Avoid Over-styling

The rise of the man bun over the past couple of years brought the term 'traction alopecia' into the mainstream and women everywhere freaked out because they have been wearing their hair up forever! Traction alopecia is a form of gradual hair loss which occurs when the hair is constantly pulled e.g. tight braiding, tight ponytails (and man buns!).

Overuse of heated styling products like flat irons and curlers can also cause damage to the hair which can cause it to break and fall. If you must fry your hair, make sure to use a heat protection spray and try not to do it every day.

Lots of styling products like gels, mousses and hair sprays can also cause hair to become brittle and dry which can lead to breakage and hair loss. It's a good idea to keep products to a minimum and, as much as possible, use natural products and make sure to wash them out at the end of the day – definitely don't try to brush them out! There are more healthy-hair tips in earlier chapters.

Use Good Quality Haircare Products

As alluded to earlier, natural is best when it comes to your hair. Natural and organic haircare products can be more expensive than their chemical counterparts, but if you're worried about hair loss, they are a must. The mainstream chemical-laden shampoos and conditioners can cause irritation; dry and strip the hair; and can harm the hair and scalp with long-term use. For whatever reason, if you can't bring yourself to switch to natural and organic haircare products, at least get some good quality products from your hairdresser—the supermarket stuff is simply junk food for your hair.

Avoid Emotional and Physical Stress

Yes, I know, easier said than done. Avoiding all kinds of stress has many health benefits including keeping your hair on your head. Unless you're already susceptible to hair loss, you're unlikely to experience hair loss as a result of the minor hitches and glitches of everyday life. However, as we saw in earlier chapters, hair loss can be caused by the type of emotional stress experienced during divorce or when a loved one dies.

Physical stress occurs during an illness or injury when your body is too busy keeping you alive to bother about growing your hair. Being diagnosed with a serious illness or being in a bad car accident can certainly cause your body enough physical stress to cause hair fall. Be proactive and seek help from your GP to get better when you need to ... it may just help you hold onto your hair.

Some forms of hair loss are hereditary, and in women, the tendency for hair loss to be one of your body's response mechanisms can also be inherited. So if you have this tendency in your family and you are wanting to try to prevent your hair from falling victim (pun not intended!), then take these tips on board and be kind to your hair while also making the time to keep yourself in good health.

And remember, forewarned is often forearmed!

Is There a Cure?

Of course, if there was a real cure I would have already written a book about it! The harsh fact of the matter is that while there are plenty of scientists doing great work to find a cure for hair loss, and there is some hope, there are only a few options and trials that you could potentially latch onto.

Here I have covered some of the common solutions that many report *do* make a difference.

Platelet Rich Plasma

Another day, another miracle cure! One of the latest grains of hope to come out of the scientific community is platelet rich plasma (or PRP) for hair loss. It sounds very sci-fi and very promising and many have jumped on the bandwagon. To save you from another potentially money wasting fate, I have done all the research for you on PRP—what it is and how it works.

What is it?

If you remember back to biology class you'll probably recall that blood is made up of plasma, red blood cells, white blood cells and platelets. Whilst you may recall platelets as being responsible for clotting, what you may not know is that they also contain hundreds of proteins called 'growth factors'. Growth factors are capable of stimulating cellular growth, proliferation, healing and cellular differentiation (sounds promising for hair regrowth, doesn't it?). After undergoing a couple of harvests (having blood taken), patients undergoing PRP are re-injected with their own blood which has been improved to contain a concentration of their own platelets—roughly five times the typical baseline level.

The theory behind this process is that the more platelets in the blood, the more growth factors in the blood; and the more growth factors in the blood, the more cellular activity; and the more cellular activity, the more hair will grow! Simple, right? Well...

Does PRP Regrow Hair?

First, let's get one thing straight. NOTHING can regrow hair where there is no hair. The only way you can have hair again where there is no hair is to take active hair follicles from somewhere else on the body or scalp and transplant them to somewhere where there is no hair. This is why hair transplants are widely used to increase the amount of hair on the head.

The best that PRP can do is to thicken up existing hair. So when PRP treatment experts say it can *regrow* hair what they actually mean is, it can make fine (thin) hair that is already there into hair that may be in better health and therefore may grow stronger and thicker.

There have been a few scientific studies on the effectiveness of PRP treatments for hair regrowth but they have been quite basic and only utilised small sample sizes.

One very small study carried out on 5 males by the Plastic and Reconstructive Surgery Department at the University of Rome in 2014, found a mean increase in total hair density of 27.7 (number of hairs/cm^2) following PRP treatments. This increase was noted after 3 months.

Another small study with 11 participants was published in the Journal of Cutaneous and Aesthetic Surgery in 2014. In this trial there was also evidence of an increase in the density of hair with an average mean gain of 22.09 follicular units per cm^2. Less than in the previous trial mentioned. However, in this study a slowing of hair loss was also noted.

Is PRP Suitable for Women?

There would seem to be no reason why it wouldn't be suitable for women; however, it is worth noting that the earlier the therapy is applied, the more likely it is to be successful. As mentioned earlier, the follicles must still be active for the PRP treatment to work.

Also, bear in mind the clinical research we were able to find has been based on extremely small sample sizes and there were no women involved in these studies.

A word of caution: PRP treatments increase the growth of cells which it comes into contact with. This means that if there are any skin cancer cells in the vicinity, these too could be affected in a way which could make them also grow faster.

What Is the Process?

PRP treatment first involves having blood taken (usually from the arm). This blood is then put into a machine that separates out the platelets from the other blood cells via a process called centrifugation. These isolated platelets are then added back to the patient's own blood in a much higher concentration than it would normally be and re-injected subcutaneously (just under the skin surface), via mesotherapy, back into the same patient.

This is repeated in 3-4 treatments over a 5-6-week period. Each treatment takes up to 90 minutes. If there are signs of good results in a given subject, then the treatment will need to be repeated every 3-6 months for the treatment to continue producing a benefit. To clarify, PRP treatments for hair loss must be ongoing to remain effective. Once the treatment stops, the decline in hair thickness will pick up where it left off.

It is also worth bearing in mind that over time, the hair around the treated area may also become sparse and new areas may need treatment. Thus, once hair loss has advanced to a certain level, PRP treatments may need to cease to avoid an uneven result.

Since the 1970s PRP has been used in various clinical applications, including cardiology, sports medicine, cosmetic surgery and pain management. However, it is only recently that it has begun to be associated with hair regrowth. Although plenty of companies suggest that they have had great success with PRP for hair regrowth, there is an obvious lack of solid scientific evidence, with the exception of the two very small studies I have mentioned here.

So while there are some positive indications that PRP could be useful in the treatment of hair loss, it is worth remembering that it is a fairly new application of the therapy, and while it can help in some cases, it is not going to be suitable for everyone. Furthermore, above all it will not *regrow* hair where there is no hair.

Hair Plucking

A huge amount of buzz has arisen relating to a possible breakthrough in follicle regeneration. It is centred on the counterintuitive idea that plucking hairs could actually result in more hair growth. So, is this true? Should we all be grabbing the tweezers and intentionally balding ourselves in the pursuit of a full head of hair?

The Study

Scientists studied the regeneration of hair follicles in response to patterned hair plucking in mice. They discovered that by plucking 200 hairs in a specific pattern in a limited area, more than 1,000 hairs grew back in their place, as well as in nearby regions. Interestingly, if the hairs were plucked from random spots or over larger areas, this regeneration did not occur.

Why Did This Happen?

Scientists believe that the affected hair follicles were able to communicate with other follicles and send them a type of distress signal. Those follicles then responded by regenerating as much as five times the amount of replacement hair.

This phenomenon is similar to the way that bacteria functions. Bacteria are able to communicate with each other through a chemical signalling system called quorum sensing. They use this to detect when their numbers are strong enough to achieve their objective.

Can This Help Hair Loss?

This finding is a big breakthrough for science, but unfortunately not a big breakthrough for hair loss yet, even though it may sound like one.

According to lead researcher, Cheng-Ming Chuong M.D., Ph.D. of the Keck School of Medicine, Dept. of Pathology, University of Southern California, more studies are needed to determine whether these findings may be able to contribute to combating hair loss in the future.

Although many hair loss bloggers may be touting this study as the breakthrough we have all been waiting for, it seems to be a bit of a red herring. Still, here's hoping that these findings lead to further study which may provide that breakthrough we're all ready for!

Minoxidil

Minoxidil is a topical treatment that is widely used for the treatment of hair loss. It generally comes in two different strengths, 5% for men and 2% for women. It can be effective in helping promote hair growth in both males and females with androgenic alopecia.

There is certainly evidence that Minoxidil works to regrow hair and it is approved by the US Food and Drug Administration for use in the treatment of androgenic hair loss.

Amongst other things, Minoxidil is a vasodilator, that is, it opens up blood vessels to increase the blood flow through them. This in turn increases the availability of oxygen and nutrients to the area to which it is applied—in this case the hair follicle.

While I have read that exactly how Minoxidil works to regrow hair is not completely understood, the vasodilation action would certainly seem to be one plausible explanation. The type of hair regrowth experienced, however, is often very fine and not of the quality of the original hair lost.

There are a few important factors to note with Minoxidil use. Firstly, it seems to work best on areas of sparse hair, not areas of complete baldness. In addition, it would appear that it has its greatest effect on younger men who have experienced their hair loss within 5 years. Finally, the most important factor to note is that if Minoxidil works, it only works while the user continues to use it. Once the user stops, the hair is shed again.

This is probably one of the most disappointing aspects of this otherwise wonderful hair regrowth treatment. It is quite expensive and to find that you have to become attached to using it, can be problematic.

Products containing Minoxidil are available all over the world as an over-the-counter product.

Propecia

You may have heard of a product called Propecia, also sold as Proscar (aka finasteride). This is a drug taken orally for the treatment of pattern baldness in men.

Propecia in not approved by the American FDA for use by women because, among other things, it is known to cause birth defects on the unborn male foetus. The drug's label warns that women who are pregnant or may become pregnant must not even *handle* this drug under any circumstances.

Propecia works by decreasing the concentration of Dihydrotestosterone (DHT) in the blood and therefore the scalp.

An elevated level of DHT, known colloquially as 'bad testosterone', is associated with benign prostatic hyperplasia (enlarged prostate), prostate cancer and you guessed it, a reduction in healthy hair follicles.

So, while it would seem to be an open and shut case, hormones are a delicate and tricky thing and there are not a lot of reliable ways to manipulate them without causing other problems.

For example, some men experience sexual side effects such as erectile dysfunction and decreased libido when taking finasteride.

As is required under USA federal law, in order to gain FDA approval for use in treating hair loss, controlled clinical studies must be carried out to prove efficacy. Hence, several clinical studies have been performed on men using Propecia. The results, while positive, are not overwhelming.

Low doses of finasteride taken over five years have been seen to reduce the concentration of DHT in the blood and, therefore, have a positive effect on both preventing hair loss and triggering regrowth. However, the amount of improvement is fairly small. Two-percent regrowth was the average, and that was in men with mild to moderate hair loss.

According to Section 14.2 of the FDA label for Propecia, a small study was also carried out on post-menopausal women. Over a period of twelve months, some 137 women were treated with Propecia or a placebo. At the end of the trial they were unable to demonstrate any improvement in hair count, as reported by the women themselves, nor was it visible in before and after photos.

Finasteride isn't the baldness cure some would have us believe. You can find more information about the studies that were carried out in Section 14 of the FDA label which you can find on the FDA website.

Given that Propecia is not recommended for women, you may be interested to know that a study by Harvard Medical School in 2003, found that consuming soy products and/or black tea did inhibit the production of DHT, so maybe allow yourself that extra soy tea?

The Trichologist

A book on hair loss would not be complete without mentioning trichologists.

Trichology is a para-medical, scientific discipline describing the study of the hair and scalp. A Trichologist therefore is someone who specialises in diagnosing and treating hair and scalp problems.

Some trichologists come from a hair-dressing background, some from completely unrelated backgrounds, and I know many who have come from a nursing or paramedical background.

The important thing to know is that if you are not having great success discussing your hair loss or your thinning hair with a doctor, a trichologist is an option you should consider.

You will find it easy to track down a trichologist in your area, but first, a few words of caution and advice.

Like any non-medical 'treatment' or practitioner, there are all sorts of charlatans out there! It is not uncommon for a hairdresser to add an extra certificate in trichology practice to a hairdressing certificate, nor for a large multi-national hair loss clinic to headline a trichologist on staff as part of a sales pitch.

There are several paths to so-called trichology certification, from a one-day in-house training course to years spent in a recognised academic training program, so it is important that you establish the credentials of the trichologist you are considering for your treatment.

You will find that a comprehensively trained, professional and certified trichologist will have a high level of knowledge and will be competent in diagnosing and solving many hair loss issues—including for women.

It is definitely worth thoroughly checking out the trichologists in your area before allowing anyone to take on board your health or your money. Here are a number of questions worth asking:

- Ask what qualifications a trichologist has
- Check their website for evidence of training and certification
- Ensure they are a member of an official trichology association such as the World Trichology Society, The Trichological Society (UK) or The International Association of Trichologists (Australia)
- Ask to speak to a previous client. While that may sound like one step too far, you will find that any quality trichology professional will be only too happy to put you in contact with a previous client or two, since they have nothing to hide

Once you have found a professionally qualified trichologist, you will no doubt find that you are in good hands.

Hair Fibres— a Cosmetic Solution

The secret to instantly thicker hair is to shake in a hair fibre concealer.

What Exactly Are Hair Fibres?

Hair fibres are tiny hair-like micro fibres that come in a variety of hair colours. They are added to fine, thin and thinning hair to instantly make hair thicker. The latest technology hair fibres are made from cotton.

How do you apply hair fibres?

Simply shake onto dry hair and lightly blend in with finger tips to disperse the fibres down the hair shaft. They can be applied to hair following the addition of the usual styling products. As long as the hair is dry the fibres will cling.

They stay in place in wind and light rain until they are washed out. Some people like to use a hair spray to keep their style in place and no doubt this can help keep the fibres in place, but generally you will find that cotton hair fibres don't require any fixing spray. In fact, if you find hair fibres that do require a fixing spray then you are probably looking at the old keratin technology.

How do they work?

Hair fibres are slightly electrostatically charged and they cling to dry hair, surrounding the hair shaft itself to make it appear up to ten times thicker. The best and most recent technology hair fibres on the market today are made from cotton. The reason cotton hair fibres are considered the most superior hair fibres is because cotton is colour fast and also non-irritating. In addition, cotton hair fibres have a far superior cling factor. They are more readily electrostatic (think pulling a jumper over your head). This creates the instant cling factor.

Some of the old technology hair fibres are made from animal fur or animal hair, which require a lot of chemical and antibiotic treatments to make them suitable for human use. These products are then claimed to mimic the type of keratin found in human hair.

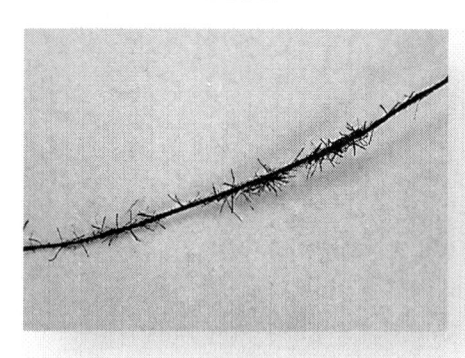

The problem with the old technology is that the chemical concoction is water soluble and is known to dissolve in sweat, and when it dissolves, it turns green.

Many people report having the look of something green in their hair when standing in the sun.

Here is a hair magnified 25 times showing cotton hair fibres clinging to the hair shaft thus demonstrating how hair fibres can make hair appear up to ten times thicker

So I recommend you look out for the latest technology products that are made from cotton.

The old technology hair fibres can also be sticky, clump on the scalp and are known to be itchy.

Cotton hair fibres are 100% natural and are actually derived from the cotton plant. Since we wear cotton next to our skin every day, we already know it is non-irritating.

Can they be detected once applied?

The great thing about cotton hair fibres is that they look completely natural. They have been designed to blend in with natural hair.

Cotton hair building fibres are never detectable if applied correctly. You can get within an inch of someone's hair after they have applied hair fibres and you won't be able to see them.

They come in a range of colours, so as long as the colour chosen is close to the hair colour, they will be completely undetectable.

Don't worry, your secret is safe!

How do I know which colour to choose?

Always choose the colour closest to your root colour. If in doubt or between two colour choices, choose the darker option. Dark roots are more flattering on someone with thinning hair.

What if my roots are grey?

In this case, choose the colour you are dying your hair. One great side effect of cotton hair fibres is that they cover up the grey root colour and many ladies find they get another week or so out of their hair colour!

Are there any side effects?

No. Unless someone is allergic to cotton. There are usually trace elements of a few other ingredients which are combined with cotton to ensure that the fibres fall onto the hair and are not flying around in the air, and also to colour them. But it is very rare for someone to experience any negative side effects.

Will it work on completely bald spots?

Hair fibres are designed to cling to hair—even the finest, almost invisible hair. So for a complete bald spot, the best option is to grow your hair over it if you can and then thicken up the hair that is covering the bald spot using hair fibres. That will help to disguise it.

Why haven't I heard of hair fibres before?

In my day-to-day business helping women with hair loss, I get asked this question so often. The answer is simply that no one had made a product like this for women - until recently. There are a lot of keratin based products on the market for men, and many of those put the obligatory picture of a woman on their website showing a female using the product, but the reality is, these products were designed by men for men!

In 2013, a group of women got together and designed hair fibres for women—in women's hair colours and with women in mind. That brought about the development of BOOSTnBLEND hair fibres for women.

Is it easy to adjust to wearing hair fibres?

Cotton hair fibres stay in place no matter what you do – even while you sleep. I often experience high wind on the weekends on a boat. The first time, I headed straight for the on-board toilet mirror to check my hair, and even after half an hour of high wind, the fibres hadn't budged!

The photos below (shown here in a variety of hair loss situations) will give you an idea of what you can expect after one application. As you can see, they can make an enormous difference.

These before and after photos show the instant results attained following one shake-in application of BOOSTnBLEND cotton hair fibres for women

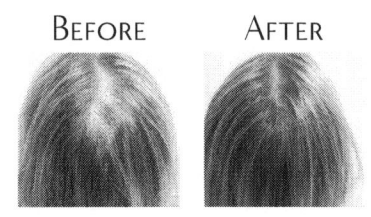

BEFORE AFTER

Many women find their crown is the first place to thin out. Hair fibres can fill this area in very well.

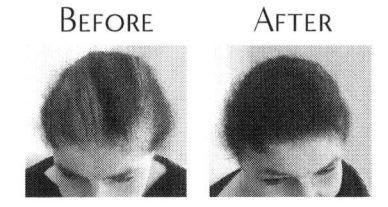

BEFORE AFTER

Even for advanced hair loss in women, a single application of hair fibres can make a real difference

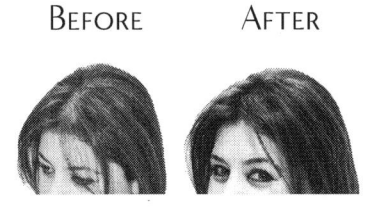

BEFORE AFTER

Another common presentation is the widening part with visible thinning in the front. A simple shake of hair fibres can completely obscure the scalp and create instantly thicker hair.

Conclusion

I sincerely hope that this book has given you some food for thought. In particular, some useful tips and tricks as well as some ideas on what could be contributing to your thinning hair.

I have covered many of the most common causes of thinning hair in women. There are undoubtedly others, such as metabolic disorders and causes related to medication. I have deliberately stayed away from those as hair loss is likely to be part of a range of symptoms which you should be discussing with your general practitioner.

Even so, general practitioners are seeing more and more women with hair loss. As mentioned earlier, a recent study in the UK reported that 64% of the GPs surveyed said they had seen an increase in the number of women with hair loss in the preceding five years.

So, we are not alone. In fact, we are in very good company. I am often astounded by the number of female celebrities suffering from visibly thinning hair and like anyone who hasn't yet found the right solution, the problem is there for all the world to see.

There are many things you can do to disguise this unexpected problem. For some of us, the problem will go away as unexpectedly as it arrived; yet for others, including me, we will have this for the rest of our lives.

I have certainly thickened up my hair in the past few years by getting to the root causes (for me, as you know by now, there was more than one cause) and reversing the damage. While I don't have the perfectly thick hair I once had, with the help of the remedies, tips, tricks and cover-up solutions contained in this very book, absolutely not a single person knows my secret, unless I choose to make it known (or they read this book and look me up!).

I hope and pray for each of you that you will find some of these ideas will work for you. Even a simple change of habit in the way you treat your hair each day, covered in earlier chapters, can vastly improve your hair.

While we seem to believe our hair is our crowning glory, and while I'm certainly all about helping women to regain some of that glory and the resulting confidence, I also suggest we keep our hair and our appearance in perspective.

No matter what, *the you* on the inside is much more important than *the you* on the outside. I find that people who are beautiful on the inside radiate beauty on the outside.

I think we all know this instinctively, and it's so easy to get carried away with worry about our hair—and I am certainly guilty of that myself!

But let's just remember—as Audrey Hepburn once famously said: 'The true beauty of a woman is reflected in her soul.'

So while we are working on improving our hair health, let's not lose sight of what's really important.

If you have found this book helpful, please pass it on to help someone else. Help get the word out there and let other women know that they don't have to suffer in silence, as a lot of women have told me they were doing. Use the hashtag #thinhairfat when spreading the word and ultimately help give that confidence back to more women.

I wish you health, happiness and of course, great hair days !

Bambi

References

Birch, M., Messenger, J., & Messenger, A. (2001). Hair density, hair diameter and the prevalence of female pattern hair loss. *British Journal of Dermatology*, 144(2), 297-304.

CalmClinic. (2015). How Stress and Anxiety Can Cause Hair Loss, from http://www.calmclinic.com/anxiety/symptoms/hair-loss accessed 29 September, 2015.

Darrow, J. A, (2013). Finasteride as an FDA-Approved Baldness Remedy: Is It Effective? From http://blogs.harvard.edu/billofhealth/2013/01/31/finasteride-as-an-fda-approved-baldness-remedy-is-it-effective/ Accessed May 2103.

Deloche, C., Bastien, P., Chadoutaud, S., Galan, P., Bertrais, S., Hercberg, S., & de Lacharrière, O. (2007). Low iron stores: a risk factor for excessive hair loss in non-menopausal women. *European Journal of Dermatology*, 17(6), 507-512.

Deville, Lauren (2014) Ferritin and Hair Loss. Website. http://www.drlaurendeville.com Accessed May 2016.

Dye, R. H. (1992). Nutrient composition for preventing hair loss: Google Patents.

Gilhar, A., Etzioni, A., & Paus, R. (2012). Alopecia Areata. *New England Journal of Medicine*, 366(16), 1515-1525. doi: doi:10.1056/NEJMra1103442.

Gilhar, A., Keren, A., Shemer, A., d'Ovidio, R., Ullmann, Y., & Paus, R. (2013). Autoimmune Disease Induction in a Healthy Human Organ: A Humanized Mouse Model of Alopecia Areata. *J Invest Dermatol*, 133(3), 844-847. doi: http://www.nature.com/jid/journal/v133/n3/suppinfo/jid2012365s1.html

Girman, C., Rhodes, T., Lilly, F., Guo, S., Siervogel, R., Patrick, D., & Chumlea, W. (1998). Effects of self-perceived hair loss in a community sample of men. *Dermatology* (Basel, Switzerland), 197(3), 223-229.

Gizlenti, S., & Ekmekci, T. (2014). The changes in the hair cycle during gestation and the post=partum period. *Journal of the European Academy of Dermatology and Venereology*, 28(7), 878-881.

Hadshiew, I. M., Foitzik, K., Arck, P. C., & Paus, R. (2004). Burden of hair loss: stress and the underestimated psychosocial impact of telogen effluvium and androgenetic alopecia. *Journal of Investigative Dermatology*, 123(3), 455-457.

Hughes E. CW. Telogen Effluvium. Website. http://emedicine.medscape.com/article/1071566-overview. Accessed 8 April 2011.

Hunt, N., & McHale, S. (2005). The psychological impact of alopecia. *British Medical Journal*, 331(7522), 951.

Ishida, W., Makino, T., & Shimizu, T. (2011). Severe hair loss of the scalp due to a hair dye containing para phenylenediamine. ISRN dermatology, 2011.

Jacques, J. (2006). Micronutrition for the weight loss surgery patient: Matrix Medical Communications.

Kaufman, K. D., Olsen, E. A., Whiting, D., Savin, R., DeVillez, R., Bergfeld, W., Price VH, Van Neste D, Roberts JL, Hordinsky M, Shapiro J, Binkowitz B, Gormley GJ. (1998). Finasteride in the treatment of men with androgenetic alopecia. *Journal of the American Academy of Dermatology*, 39(4), 578-589.

Kellenberger, D. (2011). Understanding Hair Loss after Bariatric Surgery, from https://www.drdkim.net/ask-the-dietitian/understanding-hair-loss-after-bariatric-surgery Accessed 2 September 2015.

Kligman, A. M. (1961). Pathologic dynamics of human hair loss: I. telogen effluvium. *Archives of Dermatology*, 83(2), 175-198. doi: 10.1001/archderm.1961.01580080005001

Leigh, W. (2013). Hair loss...on a woman? It's happening to increasing numbers of us - and it eats away at your femininity like an acid. The Daily Mail Australia. Retrieved from http://www.dailymail.co.uk/femail/article-2344666/Hair-loss--woman-Its-happening-increasing-numbers-eats-away-femininity-like-acid.html Accessed 15 June 2014.

Merck & Co., Inc (2012) Propecia: *Highlights of Prescribing Information*. Retrieved from http://www.accessdata.fda.gov/drugsatfda_docs/label/2012/020788s020s021s023lbl.pdf. Accessed May 2016.

Mirzoyev, S. A., Schrum, A. G., Davis, M. D., & Torgerson, R. R. (2014). Lifetime Incidence Risk of Alopecia Areata Estimated at 2.1% by Rochester Epidemiology Project, 1990-2009. *Journal of Investigative Dermatology*, 134(4), 1141-1142.

MJB. (2014). My Disastrous Experience Taking Biotin Supplements for Hair Growth, from http://blackgirllonghair.com/2014/02/my-results-of-taking-biotin/ Accessed 28 April 2015.

Mubki, T., Rudnicka, L., Olszewska, M., & Shapiro, J. (2014). Evaluation and diagnosis of the hair loss patient: part II. Trichoscopic and laboratory evaluations. *Journal of the American Academy of Dermatology*, 71(3), 431.e431-431.e411. doi: 10.1016/j.jaad.2014.05.008.

Nutrition Review (2015) Reversing Age-Related Hair Loss and Restoring Healthy Hair Growth in Men and Women from http://nutritionreview.org/2015/08/reversing-age-related-hair-loss-and-restoring-healthy-hair-growth-in-men-and-women/ Accessed May 2016.

Oliver, D. (2015). Why You Should Be Cautious Of Taking Biotin For Your Hair, Skin & Nails, The Huffington Post. Retrieved from http://www.huffingtonpost.com/2013/09/30/biotin-hair-skin-nails_n_4016804.html Accessed 28 April 2015

Olsen, E. A., Whiting, D. A., Savin, R., Rodgers, A., Johnson-Levonas, A. O., Round, E., Rotonda J, Kaufman, K. D. Global photographic assessment of men aged 18 to 60 years with male pattern hair loss receiving finasteride 1 mg or placebo. *Journal of the American Academy of Dermatology*, 67(3), 379-386. doi: 10.1016/j.jaad.2011.10.027.

Orme, S., Cullen, D., & Messenger, A. (1999). Diffuse female hair loss: are androgens necessary? *British Journal of Dermatology*, 141, 521-523.

Price, V. H. (1999). Treatment of Hair Loss. *New England Journal of Medicine*, 341(13), 964-973. doi: doi:10.1056/NEJM199909233411307.

Rakowska, A., Slowinska, M., Kowalska-Oledzka, E., Warszawik, O., Czuwara, J., Olszewska, M., & Rudnicka, L. (2012). Trichoscopy of cicatricial alopecia. *Journal of Drugs in Dermatology*, 11(6), 753-758.

Randall, V. A., & Ebling, F. J. G. (1991). Seasonal changes in human hair growth. *British Journal of Dermatology*, 124(2), 146-151. doi: 10.1111/j.1365-2133.1991.tb00423.x.

Rudnicka, L., Olszewska, M., Rakowska, A., & Slowinska, M. (2011). Trichoscopy update 2011. *Journal of Dermatological Case Reports*, 5(4), 82-88. doi: 10.3315/jdcr.2011.1083.

Rushton, D. (1993). Management of hair loss in women. *Dermatologic Clinics*, 11(1), 47-53.

Rushton, D. (2002). Nutritional factors and hair loss. *Clinical and Experimental Dermatology*, 27(5), 396-404.

Rushton, D. (2002). Nutritional factors and hair loss. *Clinical and experimental Dermatology*, 27(5), 396-404.

Rushton, D., Norris, M., Dover, R., & Busuttil, N. (2002). Causes of hair loss and the developments in hair rejuvenation. *International Journal of Cosmetic Science*, 24(1), 17-23.

Samuels, Lawrence (2013) Maintaining a Healthy Scalp and Hair for Improved Hair Growth, *The Dermatologist* 21(6).

Retrieved from http://www.the-dermatologist.com. Accessed May 2016.

Sarah. (2015). FDA Clears Capillus In-Clinic Laser Therapy Hair Growth Device, from http://www.belgraviacentre.com/blog/category/belgravias-advice-on-the-most-well-known-hair-loss-products/ Accessed July 2015

Shapiro, J. (2013). Current Treatment of Alopecia Areata. Paper presented at the Journal of Investigative Dermatology Symposium Proceedings.

Shapiro, J., & Otberg, N. (2015). Hair Loss and Restoration. CRC Press.

Søsted, H., Agner, T., Andersen, K. E., & Menné, T. (2002). 55 cases of allergic reactions to hair dye: a descriptive, consumer complaint-based study. *Contact Dermatitis*, 47(5), 299-303.

The Trichological Society (2014). Hair/Scalp Conditions/Disorders Index 2014 from http://www.hairscientists.org. Accessed May 2016.

Trost, L. B., Bergfeld, W. F., & Calogeras, E. (2006). The diagnosis and treatment of iron deficiency and its potential relationship to hair loss. *Journal of the American Academy of Dermatology*, 54(5), 824-844.

Trüeb, R. M. (2003). Association between smoking and hair loss: another opportunity for health education against smoking? *Dermatology* (Basel, Switzerland), 206(3), 189-191. doi: 10.1159/000068894.

Whiting, D. A. (1996). Chronic telogen effluvium: increased scalp hair shedding in middle-aged women. *Journal of the American Academy of Dermatology*, 35(6), 899-906.

Williamson, D., Gonzalez, M., & Finlay, A. (2001). The effect of hair loss on quality of life. *Journal of the European Academy of Dermatology and Venereology*, 15(2), 137-139.

Wood, A. J., & Price, V. H. (1999). Treatment of hair loss. *New England Journal of Medicine*, 341(13), 964-973.